NEWBIES GUIDE TO INTERMITTENT FASTING

A Step By Step Plan To Becoming The New You

John B. Strong

DEDICATION

*For all those who have the courage
and boldness to change their
lives by changing their bodies.*

John B. Strong

TABLE OF CONTENTS

WHAT IS FASTING?

What It Is and What It Isn't

Fasting is the abstinence of all kinds of food and drink over a period of time. Fasting can be done for a day, a week, or a month – this is dependent on the needs of the individual and the goal that they want to achieve. It can be done as an absolute fast – complete abstinence or intermittent fast that involves no food for a specific time.

Fasting is an age-old practice that has been undertaken by all nationalities, whether for personal or for religious reasons. It is done to achieve a particular goal or a specific outcome.

In the religious arena, fasting is done as an act of devotion to God and to enhance spiritual growth.

There are different varieties of fasting, which makes it a lot more attractive. It should not only be considered as a method to lose weight but as a temporary activity to strengthen your focus for a particular gain. A few examples are: giving up meat during lent, abstain from social media, giving up desserts, alcohol, a meal or two, or even television.

People also fast if they have to undergo a medical procedure for various tests, surgery, and general anesthesia.

Weight loss is one of the main reasons why people fast. Many weight loss diet plans are comprised of periods of fasting. This activity has been beneficial for many persons; consequently, it is recommended in weight loss programs.

On a different side of fasting, it helps to cleanse or rid the body of toxins. Depriving the body of food and drink, meats, snacks, etc. allows the body to go through a cleansing process. Many persons are becoming more conscious of the type of food they consume, and this may be due to the illnesses that are affecting people. Consequently, many opt to do a green juice fast to become healthier. It helps the body to heal, rejuvenate, enhance mental health, reduce the risk of chronic disease, reduce inflammation, stimulate the cells, and energize the entire body.

Green juices come from green leafy vegetables, cucumbers, green apples, and celery. This type of m juice is loaded with micronutrients that are critical for cellular nutrition. Fasting on juices helps the body to absorb more nutrients, make digestion easier and less oxidative stress. The nutrients from the green juice are absorbed into the bloodstream quickly – this will cleanse the blood, liver, kidneys, and digestive tract. Many persons incorporate fasting in their weight loss program, and this will vary. The program starts with a strict regimen of reducing carbohydrates and foods that are high in calories. It is recommended that you drink a lot of water. Sweetened drinks should be avoided as they are usually high in sugar.

WHAT IS INTERMITTENT FASTING ?

Intermittent fasting involves periods of fasting ranging from 12 – 36 hours. It is not a diet; it is a different way of scheduling meals to get more benefits out of a fasting program to result in a weight reduction. Water, unsweetened tea or drinks, and black coffee are allowed during this period. The aim is to consume no more than 600 calories within two days.

The most obvious benefit of intermittent fasting is to reduce calories, which will lead to weight loss. Intermittent fasting involves alternating an average meal with a meal that is seen to have less calories. People are of the view that it will help them to lose weight faster, reduce inflammation, reduce heart disease, and overall a healthier body. Intermittent fasting increases the metabolic rate by up to 14 percent, which paves the way for the body to burn more calories.

Compared to diets, intermittent fasting is an easy program to follow, as it requires minimal adjustment in regular activity. However, care has to be taken not to eat foods that are high in calories, as this can defeat the purpose of going on an intermittent fast.

Interestingly, our bodies are designed to go without food for a specific period of time. While the body needs sleep to rest, repair, and revitalize, our organs and digestive tract need to rest as well to become more efficient. It should be noted, that allowing periods of intermittent fasting can result in anti-inflammatory responses:

Improvement in the overall gut microbiota structure.

Less dependency on insulin.

Enhancement of immune cell responsiveness.

Increase in the production of B-hydroxybutyrate compound that is involved in health disorders such as Alzheimer's, diabetes, and rheumatoid arthritis.

There is also significantly less production of cytokines, and C-reactive protein.

BENEFITS OF INTERMITTENT FASTING

More Than Meets The Eye

Weight loss is the first benefit of intermittent fasting. Carbohydrates absorbed by the body is broken down into glucose, which is used for energy or converted and stored as fat. Insulin, which is a hormone that is produced by the pancreas, enables the cells to absorb glucose. During the fast, the insulin level decreases as a result of less food intake; this causes the cells to facilitate fat burning by releasing the stored glucose as energy. If this process is repeated regularly, it will lead to weight loss.

It is best to eat fruits, vegetables, lentils, peas and beans, lean proteins, and a plant-based diet for desired results. It is not advisable to continue high-calorie foods such as sugary food and drinks in the form of ice cream, cakes, snacks, sweetened beverages, etc. and refined grains. Consideration should be given to the hours for intermittent fasting. Research has indicated that it is most effective starting earlier in the day from 7 am to 3 pm, or 10 am to 6 pm. Snacking late evening or nighttime should be avoided.

Lowers The Risk of
Type 2 Diabetes

Being overweight is contributory to Type 2 Diabetes. The weight loss program will, therefore, benefit persons who are diagnosed with this type of disease and who are predisposed to it. Losing weight will also protect the individual from developing diabetes-related complications like neuropathy, retinopathy, liver damage, kidney damage, heart disease.

Lowers Blood Pressure

Studies that have been published in the European Journal have indicated that intermittent fasting has a positive effect by reducing high blood pressure. It is imperative to have a healthy blood pressure to prevent heart disease, stroke, and kidney disease. The reduction in blood pressure will only last as long as the intermittent fast. Once the practice comes to an end, the blood pressure readings will likely return to the original levels.

Improved Heart Health

Less consumption of fats and sugar during intermittent fasting will lead to a healthier lifestyle, such as improved cardiovascular health, reduced cholesterol, and triglycerides that are linked to heart disease. The reduction of insulin levels causes less cardiovascular risk, such as congestive heart failure. This reduction is particularly significant to persons with Type 2 diabetes since they are more likely to be affected by heart disease.

Improved Brain Health

There is the possibility that intermittent fasting may cause neuronal autophagy to take place, which is the growth of brain cells – which offers protection for the brain.

Lower Cancer Risk

Obesity is viewed as a risk factor for cancer. Losing weight during the intermittent fast is an excellent way of reducing biological factors that are associated with cancer, insulin levels, and inflammation.

Increased Cell Production

Intermittent fast provides a period of rest for the body. During this time, there is an increase of autophagy – a detoxification process to clean out cells that are damaged. This period also allows the body to heal and get rid of waste in the cells that speeds up aging.

Increased Longevity

Intermittent fast brings about a cleansing process which allows the body to increase its resistance to age-related disease.

A good night's rest is almost a guarantee – the body is ridding itself of toxins, the digestive system is resting, the cells are being repaired, the body is beginning to feel lighter, less stress. Knowing your body is being cleansed, is a great way to experience tranquility and be at peace with yourself. Also enhancing the functioning of cells, hormones and genes.

Additional Benefits of Intermittent Fasting

A decrease in insulin levels that facilitates fat burning.

An increase in the growth hormone levels paves the way for muscle gain and fat burning.

The removal of waste from the cells and repair processes to take place, giving the body a boost in energy facilitating cellular repair.

Reduction in cholesterol levels.

Stabilization of blood sugar count and a less need for medication.

Improvement in hemoglobin A1c levels.

Improvement in the structure of genes and molecules for protection against disease and longevity.

THE 16:8 METHOD

*Plan Your Day Instead Of
The Day Planning You*

The 16:8 method has become one of the most prevalent styles of conducting a fast. It is an easy, convenient, and straightforward method to use for weight loss and to improve your overall health.

This method works by consuming food within 8 hours and abstain from food for 16 hours. It is best to consume food and drinks that are nutritious and have a low-calorie count to achieve the desired results. Having smaller meals during the 8 hours is ideal as it will help to stave off the hunger pangs, and this can be repeated frequently; however, it depends on the individual's preference. The method is considered to be more flexible for individuals of any age group, doesn't command any preparation, less restrictive, and more comfortable than other diet plans.

Health benefits to be derived from using this method includes enhanced brain function and longevity and improvement in blood sugar control.

DAILY AND WEEKLY FASTING

Short Term or Long Haul

Daily intermittent fasting is done every day, which makes it easier to form the habit of eating within the 8-hour schedule. Some persons opt to eliminate a meal or two, which makes it a little more challenging to lose the same amount of calories.

Weekly Intermittent Fasting

Weekly intermittent fasting is a great way to get started this can be done once per week. It is certainly not the way to lose a considerable number of pounds, but with consistency, they will add up over time.

THE WARRIOR DIET

The 24 Split

Ori Holmekler created the Warrior Diet diet in 2001.

This type of fasting is a 20-hour window in which very little is eaten, such as fruits and raw vegetables. The 4 hours that is left is the time to eat. During the 4 hours, it is in a person's best interest to consume as many vegetables, proteins, healthy fats, and carbohydrates for energy.

The challenge with this fast is the lack of nutrients such as fiber.

Persons may run the risk of not consuming enough nutrients and fiber with this fast. Lack of nutrients and fiber can harm the digestive and immune system. It may also increase the risk of diseases such as cancer.

OMAD

*One Meal A Day Keeps
the Fat Away*

The One Meal A Day fasting diet is an extreme diet plan method of losing weight. The One Meal A Day fast requires a person to eat one meal per day and fast for 23 hours. It is also referred to as the 23:1. During this 1hour period, it is best to have a nutritious meal packed with all the vitamins and minerals. Many opt not to eat or drink anything that has a high-calorie content. The fast is broken at dinner and continues until the following evening. It is advisable to have as much water as possible to keep the system hydrated.

GOAL SETTING AND TIPS

*A Goal Without A Plan
is Just A Dream*

First of all, the individual has to decide carefully on the purpose and objective of fasting, which involves losing a few pounds and dieting. Below are a number of factors that should be taken into consideration:

How critical is this to my health? Am I feeling unhealthy? Am I presently overweight? Am I at risk for developing heart disease, Type II diabetes, or other related diseases? Do I want to lose a few extra pounds to stay in shape and keep fit?

Why do I want to lose weight?

If your answer is, "I want to be healthier," then you may need to ask yourself again, "why do I need to be healthier?" Wanting to be healthier can be used as the motivating factor in losing weight. Maybe it is to build my immune system, which will stave off chronic illnesses and diseases and even the common cold. Living healthier means a better lifestyle and an inexpensive or no medical bill.

How many pounds do I want to lose?

10, 15, 20, 50 pounds…. this is dependent on my present weight. How long will it take me to lose those extra pounds?

Is fasting the best way to lose weight?

Do I need to lose a lot of pounds, or do I want to maintain my weight? With a packed daily schedule, consideration has to be given to the method that will work best. Should I consider exercise?

What is the best fasting method for me?

Do I want to do an absolute fast by keeping away from all food and drinks for a defined period and go on a water diet or use an intermittent fast method?

Can I use this method effectively and efficiently?

With a busy schedule, will I be able to use this method effectively and efficiently.

Does it involve a lot of preparation time?

Am I going to have the time to make smoothies, fruit, or vegetable juices?

Is it cost-effective?

Will I be able to afford to purchase the necessary fruits,

vegetables, and nuts for my new diet plan? Is it going to be cheaper or more expensive than regular food? No doubt, it will be less expensive due to the reduced food intake.

When do I want to begin?

Do I want to begin now? Do I wait until my vacation? How crucial is it that I need to start immediately?

Is it flexible for my lifestyle?

If I am consuming a lot more fluids in my diet, will I be able to continue doing my sales job. Checking daily appointments are meetings in the office, out of office?, Will I be driving or taking the bus or train? What is the weather like? Is it a rainy or sunny day? No doubt, a cold winter's day demands more frequent trips to the bathroom. If I am in an office setting, am I near enough to a bathroom.

Should I work along with a Dietitian?

Perhaps it is best to work with a Dietitian who will encourage and guide you on the foods to eat as well as keep a check on the progress of the weight loss program. The Dietitian will provide expert advice on the nutritional needs based on your age, weight, and lifestyle. Not every diet is for everybody ...the Dietitian will recommend the best diet plan with the recommended calories to make the plan a success.

Tips that will enhance the benefits of intermittent fasting

It is best to keep hydrated by drinking lots of water, herbal teas, and drinks that are not loaded with sugar.

Thinking of food will be at the forefront of the mind – it is best to get distracted by using the time to watch a movie, plays, catch up on work, or hang out with friends.

During a fast, the energy level will reduce – it is best to avoid strenuous activities. Anything light and relaxing, e.g., yoga, will be beneficial.

Reduced calories in the fasting period should be nutritious and rich in protein, fiber, and healthy fats. Peas, beans, eggs, fish, nuts, and avocados should be included in the meals.

Aim for foods that are filling but with a low-calorie count: raw vegetables, fruits with a high water content such as melon and grapes.

Avoid using salad dressing and sugary condiments. Aim for herbs, vinegar, and garlic as these are low in calories yet flavorful and will help to reduce the hunger pangs.

Dangers of Intermittent Fasting

Discipline has to be exercised not to splurge on non-fast days as this can easily lead to adverse effects such as weight gain. Fasting can cause an increase in stress hormone and cortisol, which increases the desire for food. Two common side effects of intermittent fasting are binge eating and overeating.

Failure to drink plenty of water or fluids can lead to dehydration. Stay hydrated, consume lots of water, this will energize the body, speed up the metabolic rate, and flush out waste.

Going for walks, meditate, read – above all, keep the mind active as much as possible.

ALTERNATE DAY FASTING

Or The 5:2 Diet

This fast involves generally eating on five days and fast two days, i.e., eating low-calorie meals, e.g., salads and soups. The main goal of this fast is to reduce calorie intake by 25 percent, e.g., if the regular meals for a day is 1000 calories in total, on fast days, it should be 250.

This diet focuses on the calories on the two fast days, perfect for persons who are not bent on losing lots of pounds but instead want to keep that 'figure' or just essential maintenance. Some people will find this diet more satisfying as they won't be missing out all the time. Care should be taken; however, to eat healthy meals during the five days so that they can benefit from both high and low-calorie meals. Dark green leafy vegetables and salads should be a significant component in all meals. It will add fiber and bulk to the meal and help persons to feel more satisfied. Small portions of protein should be added to the meals, e.g., lean meat, peas and beans, tofu, eggs.

BREAKING THE FAST

The proper way to end a fast

Due care has to be taken to end a fast properly. If it is done the wrong way, it can cause the stomach to feel uncomfortable, bloated, and upset. Certain foods should be eaten to ease the body back into a regular diet gently. It is best not to overwhelm the digestive system; it is recommended to have foods in small portions as this will make it easily digestible. Below are a few tips:

Do not break fasts with a feast.

At the beginning or during the fast, some persons may feel unwell, do not continue, seek professional advice. Persons who have diabetes or suffering from other medical conditions should not go on a fast unless they have proper medical supervision. Try to eat as much protein as possible. Consume nourishing foods full of fiber on non-fast days.

Drink Fluids

During the fast, it is recommended that a lot of water should be consumed to keep hydrated. As you come towards the end of the fast, it is best to start drinking fruit juices, smoothies, milk. These beverages will be gentle on the stomach and will provide the nutrition that the body needs, such as potassium, fiber, manganese, and copper. Sugary drinks should be avoided at this stage.

Eat Dried Fruits

Excellent fruits to provide the body with natural sugars, carbohydrates, and micronutrients and fiber, e.g., raisins and dates.

Healthy Foods

Consume soups, or have very light broth. Focus on having lean protein, fruits, vegetables, nuts, and grains. Aim for a balanced diet - foods high in fiber, vitamins, minerals. Eating these will help to keep the blood sugar levels stable and prevent nutritional deficiencies.

CLOSING MOTIVATION

Never Give Up and Never Give In

Now that we have gone over the different methodologies to burn off that unwanted weight it's time to take action. That's right, it's time to roll up your sleeves and get out there and "work hard" to get the fat off and to keep it off. No more contemplating what you'll do, you have a solid game plan in this book, whatever you have to do to make it happen do it. Set a daily alarm, get accountability partners to help remind you of your goals, write things down on a calendar. Whatever you have to do in order to remember when to fast and when not to fast is paramount. No one can do this for you but you, things will not change UNTIL YOU decide to change. Take a stand and plant your flag and tell yourself "enough is enough, you're going to start this plan and you're going to stick to it until you get the results you want". My mother would always say "quitters never win", well those that don't ever start don't win either. At this point you are either going to do it or you aren't, but I'm hoping that you will start a plan, and stick with it to completion. My hope is that you will use this book as a motivational tool of insight to help you achieve your goals, the clock is ticking, see you on the other side.

If you have enjoyed this book, would you be kind enough to please leave me a review on Amazon, it would be greatly appreciated.

Click here to leave a review for this book on Amazon

Thank you .